"A

Tim Ru

"I insist that every asthma patient in my practice read this book."

Paul Ehrlich, M.D., Allergist
New York City, New York

"I give a copy of *One Minute Asthma* to parents when I first make the diagnosis. It really speeds up their learning curve."

Greg Prazar, M.D., Pediatrician
Exeter, New Hampshire

"*One Minute Asthma* is authoritative and right on the mark."

Abba Terr, M.D., Allergist
San Francisco, California

"I have yet to see a better book about asthma."

G. Bradley Gascoigne III, M.D., Pediatrician
Cleveland, Ohio

"*One Minute Asthma* provides the framework for education during our initial visit. Patients review the peak flow, holding chamber and medicine sections at home before their next visit."

Larry Westby, B.S., Respiratory Therapist
Kokomo, Indiana

"Concisely covers the major points made by the NIH Expert Panel on Asthma."

Diane Schuller, M.D., Allergist
Danville, Pennsylvania

"*One Minute Asthma* is a big help for non-patients who need to learn about asthma."

JoDee Tschirhart, R.N.
Cheyenne, Wyoming

"A great resource to get family members up to speed."

Michael Welch, M.D., Allergist
San Diego, California

"I keep a copy of *One Minute Asthma* in each exam room so that parents can improve their knowledge while they wait."

Gary Brecher, M.D., Pediatrician
Rockville, Maryland

"Fathers like the '*Fighting Asthma*' story. It reduces their concern about overmedicating."

Carey Ziemer, M.D., Pediatrician
Greensboro, North Carolina

"New patients who have read a few pages of *One Minute Asthma* in the waiting room are easier to talk to than those who haven't.

Jane Purser, M.D., Allergist
Tulsa, Oklahoma

One Minute ASTHMA

What You Need to Know

Thomas F. Plaut, M.D.
Amherst, Massachusetts

NOTICE

The information in this book is general and may not apply to your specific situation.

DO NOT CHANGE YOUR MEDICINE ROUTINE WITHOUT CONSULTING YOUR DOCTOR.

In print

English edition	*480,000 copies*
Spanish edition	*65,000 copies*

Designed by Barbara Werden
Illustrated by Carla Brennan

Library of Congress Cataloging-in-Publication Data
Plaut, Thomas F., 1933-
One minute asthma: what you need to know/ Thomas F. Plaut--1996 ed.
p. cm.
ISBN 0-914625-16-0
1. Asthma--Popular works. I. Title
RC591.P53 1996
616.2'38--DC20 96-17568
CIP

Contents

Contents continued

Introduction

I wrote *One Minute Asthma* to give asthma patients the basic facts they need to know about asthma. This includes the tools and medicines used to treat it. *One Minute Asthma* is accurate, clear, concise, easy to read, and is updated regularly.

For Teenagers and Adult Patients

First you have to understand the basics of asthma. Then you can learn how to use a peak flow meter, asthma diary and home treatment plan to control it.

For Parents

You can keep your child out of the emergency room and out of the hospital. First you must learn the basics of asthma and the medicines used to treat it. After that, you and your doctor can work out a clear, diary-based plan for treating your child's asthma at home.

For Doctors

I wrote *One Minute Asthma* because busy doctors told me they wanted to teach their patients about asthma during office and emergency room visits. Each page presents a single concept or set of facts to the patient or parent. If they read while waiting to see you, you can cover more ground during the visit.

Thomas F. Plaut, M.D.
Amherst, Massachusetts
1996

You Can Control Asthma

You and your doctor should be able to work out a plan to control asthma. After you have a good plan, you will be able to:

- Run as fast and as long as anyone else.
- Attend work or school every day.
- Sleep through the night without cough or wheeze.
- Avoid urgent visits to the doctor.
- Avoid hospitalization for asthma.

If your plan does not control your asthma symptoms fully, you and your doctor need to learn more about your asthma so you can work out a better plan.

Signs of Asthma Trouble

Cough. Worse at night, after exercise, in a smoky room or in cold air.

Wheeze. A whistling noise, often heard best when breathing out.

Breathing faster than usual. Count your breathing rate for 30 seconds. Compare this to your usual rate.

Sucking in the chest skin. Look for this in between the ribs (especially in children) and at the front of the neck (especially in adults).

If you notice any one of these signs, it is time to avoid triggers and to start or increase asthma treatment.

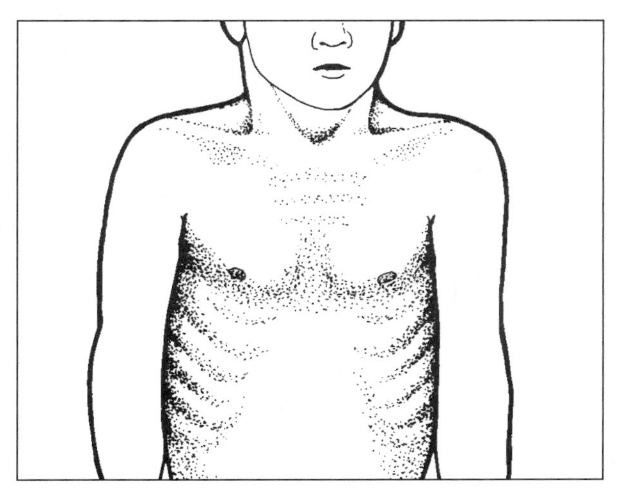

Sucking in the Chest Skin

What is Asthma?

Asthma is a long-standing (chronic) disease in which the airways are inflamed.

Asthma goes by many names: wheezy bronchitis, asthmatic bronchitis, bronchial asthma and reactive airway disease (RAD). It is often misdiagnosed as bronchitis or pneumonia.

The words "asthma episode," "asthma attack" and "asthma flare" all have the same meaning. "Airways," "bronchioles" and "windpipes" all refer to air passages in the lungs.

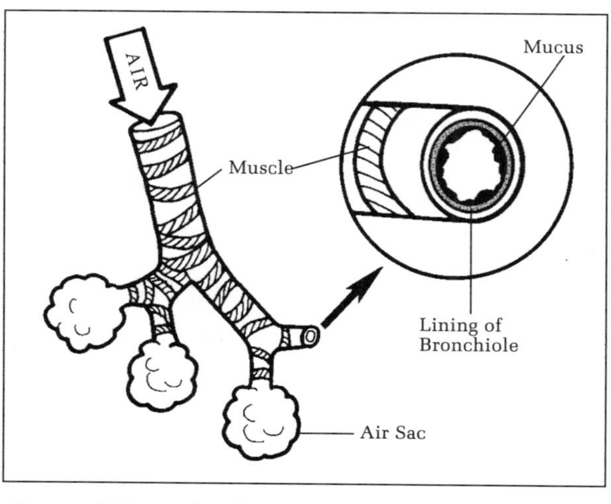

Normal Bronchiole

What Happens in the Windpipes?

People with asthma whose windpipes are inflamed react to asthma triggers such as colds, cigarette smoke and animal dander faster and more intensely than people whose windpipes are clear. During an asthma episode:

- The lining of the airways becomes more inflamed and produces more mucus. This makes the opening in the airways smaller.
- The muscles around the airways tighten, also making the opening in the airways smaller.

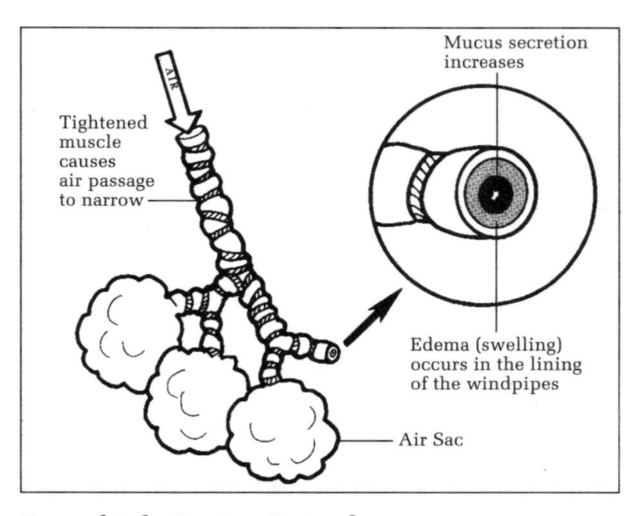

Bronchiole During Episode

Triggers

A trigger is any object, act or event that makes asthma worse.

- Exercise
- Virus infection (cold, bronchitis, pneumonia)
- Pollution like cigarette smoke, smoke from a wood stove or perfume
- Cold air
- Allergens, such as cats, dogs, mites, cockroaches, grass, mold and pollen
- Coughing, yelling and laughing
- Some medicines and chemicals

Triggers add up. Some people only develop an asthma episode if two or three triggers are present.

Avoiding Triggers

To help control asthma, avoid triggers

- Do not allow smoking in your house or car.
- Remove dustcatchers from the bedroom.
- Consider using a HEPA air filter in the bedroom.
- Consider covering heating vents with an air filter.
- Keep humidity in your house between 25 and 50 percent.
- Do not use a vaporizer or humidifier which increases the humidity above 50 percent, since mold and mites grow better in humid air.

Exercise is one trigger you should not avoid.

Exercise

Exercise is the most common trigger of asthma. Your asthma plan is not satisfactory if exercise causes:

- Cough
- A tight chest
- Wheeze

Almost every person with asthma should be fully active and be able to play any sport. With the right plan, you should be able to run as fast and as long as anyone else, except during an asthma episode.

Coughing and Asthma

Coughing may be the first sign that your asthma is not under control. People with asthma often cough:

- At night
- With exercise
- In smoky areas
- After laughing or crying
- In cold air

It can be very hard to tell an asthma cough from the cough of a regular cold. Asthma medicine will help to control an asthma cough. If the cough continues after your asthma is fully treated, a cough medicine may help.

Sinus Trouble

If your usual treatment for asthma does not clear your symptoms you may have a sinus infection.

The sinuses are air pockets in the bones of the forehead and the face. They connect to the inside of the nose by small passageways. They may become infected or inflamed by bacteria, viruses, allergens or irritants.

An inflammation may lead to infection. Taking a decongestant medicine or inhaling steriods through the nose may reduce the inflammation. This may decrease the length or the number of infections.

One sign of a sinus infection is pain when you press on the bone just above your eyebrow or on your cheek bone. Other signs of sinusitis are a severe headache or a colored discharge from your nose. Sinus infections should be treated with antibiotics.

Rinsing the nose daily with salt water may open the entrance to a sinus and help the infection drain. This may reduce the number of infections.

To make the rinsing solution, mix one half teaspoon salt in eight ounces of warm water. Then squirt the solution into your nostril with a bulb syringe or simply snort it from a saucer while pressing one nostril shut.

Medicines that May Make Asthma Worse

Aspirin and other non-steroidal anti-inflammatory drugs (NSAID) may cause asthma symptoms. About ten percent of adults with asthma have symptoms after taking these medicines. Some popular brands are Motrin, Advil, Naprosyn, Daypro and Indocin.

If you are being treated for **high blood pressure**, **angina** or **migraine headaches**, your medicine may be making your asthma worse. Cough or wheeze may appear when you start taking a medicine called a beta-blocker. This can happen even if you have never had asthma symptoms before. Some popular brands of beta-blockers are Lopressor, Corgard, Inderal and Tenormin.

People who have **glaucoma** may find their asthma worsens when they start to use beta-blocker eye drops. Using a single drop of this medicine daily may cause a cough or wheeze. Some popular brands of these eyedrops are Betoptic and Timoptic.

If these medicines are making your asthma worse ask your doctor to prescribe a type of medicine that does not cause asthma symptoms.

Inflammation of the Nose (Rhinitis)

An inflammation of the nose may trigger or prolong the symptoms of asthma. The signs of rhinitis are sneezing, a runny nose or a blocked nose.

Sometimes avoiding the triggers of rhinitis will solve the problem. If not, treatment with antihistamines, decongestants or preventer medicines (cromolyn or inhaled nasal steroids) may be helpful.

Don't Let Asthma Slow You Down

The word asthma scares a lot of people because it used to be hard to treat. Today asthma treatment is so good that most people with asthma should be able to do everything they want to do.

Certain medicines can even prevent asthma episodes from starting. They are called "preventer" medicines

You will do fine after you work out an effective plan to manage asthma with your doctor. If you and your doctor cannot achieve excellent control of your asthma, seek a consultation with an asthma specialist.

Asthma should not slow you down.

How to Choose an Asthma Doctor

You can choose a good asthma doctor by looking for these traits:

- Gives written instructions regarding dose, timing and technique for administering medicines (see Home Treatment Plan).
- Measures your peak flow or pulmonary function at each visit (see Peak Flow Meter).
- Shows you how to take your inhaled medicines and watches to check your technique— this may be done by the office staff (see Holding Chambers and Compressor-Driven Nebulizer).
- Expects you to achieve excellent control of asthma and works with you as a partner to reach this goal (see You Can Control Asthma).

Call your local hospital and ask if one of their doctors meets these standards. If not, try another hospital or call one of the organizations listed in the Resource Section.

Asthma Medicines

The two main types of asthma medicines are preventers and relievers.

Preventer medicines keep an asthma attack from happening. They are also called anti-inflammatory medicines. *They should be taken daily* by people who have signs of asthma more than one day a week. Preventer medicines are:

- Inhaled steroids. These medicines keep inflammation (swelling) of the windpipe lining from starting and reduce the inflammation that already exists in the windpipes.
- Cromolyn and nedocromil. These medicines block the asthma reaction before it starts.

Reliever medicines are mainly used to treat an attack or to prevent symptoms caused by strenuous exercise. They are also called rescue medicines. Reliever medicines are:

- Adrenaline-like medicines (albuterol, metaproterenol, pirbuterol and terbutaline). These medicines relax the muscles that have tightened around the windpipes.
- Oral steroids (prednisone, prednisolone, and methylprednisolone). They can quickly reduce the inflammation of the windpipes during an attack.
- Theophylline. This medicine relaxes the muscles that have tightened around the windpipes. It is usually used with a preventer medicine.

Inhaled Steroids

Medicine type: Preventer

Prevent asthma episodes because they decrease the overreaction of the airways to triggers and prevent inflammation of the airways.

Possible bad effects:

May cause hoarseness and a yeast infection in the mouth. To prevent these effects, use a holding chamber and rinse your mouth (and spit out) after each dose to prevent these effects.

Brand names include Vanceril, Pulmicort, Flovent, Beclovent, Azmacort and Aerobid.

The name of your medicine is: ______________.

Comment

- The bad effects of taking an inhaled steroid medicine every day are tiny compared to those of taking oral steroids every day (see Oral Steroids).
- It may take one to four weeks before an inhaled steroid medicine reaches its full effect.
- An inhaled steroid medicine is not usually helpful in treating a severe asthma attack.
- Vanceril, Flovent, Beclovent, Azmacort and Aerobid are administered by a metered-dose inhaler (MDI) with a holding chamber (see Holding Chamber).
- Pulmicort is inhaled as a powder from a breath-activated device.

Cromolyn and Nedocromil

Medicine type: Preventer

Prevent asthma episodes by blocking the inflammation of the windpipes. Also keep the muscles around the windpipes from tightening.

Possible bad effects:

Cough and bronchospasm may occur with cromolyn. Taste may sometimes be a problem with nedocromil.

The name of your medicine is: ______________.

Comment

Cromolyn (Intal) is used:

- To prevent symptoms of chronic asthma. Must be taken every day. Usually takes one to four weeks to produce full effect. Can be used for infants.
- To prevent symptoms that occur with exercise or contact with an animal, take 5 to 60 minutes before contact. The preventive effect lasts three to four hours.

Nedocromil (Tilade) is used:

- To prevent symptoms of chronic asthma in older children and adults. Takes three days for onset of effect.

For best effect, your doctor may prescribe prednisone and an inhaled adrenaline-like medicine to clear your airways for the first week of treatment. If your peak flow is not in the green zone (see Peak Flow Zones), take an adrenaline-like medicine by inhaler to dilate the airways one to three minutes before using cromolyn or nedocromil.

Adrenaline-like Medicines

Medicine type: Reliever
Dilate the windpipes.

Possible bad effects:
Shakiness or tremor and increased heart rate.

These medicines include albuterol (Proventil and Ventolin), metaproterenol (Alupent), pirbuterol (Maxair) and terbutaline (Brethaire and Bricanyl).

The name of your medicine is: ______________.

Comment

Faster, safer and more effective than theophylline for treating an attack.

Why is it better to inhale an adrenaline-like medicine than to swallow it?

- Inhaled medicines go right into the windpipes where they act. Therefore, only a very small dose is needed.
- This small dose causes less shakiness.
- Inhaled medicines usually bring relief within a few minutes. If yours doesn't work, you or your doctor will know right away that the treatment plan should be changed.
- Adrenaline-like medicines taken in pill or liquid form often require more than 20 minutes to work.

Albuterol (Ventolin) can also be inhaled as a powder from the Rotahaler, a breath-activated device.

Theophylline

Medicine type: Reliever
Dilates the windpipes.

Possible bad effects:
Hyperactivity, upset stomach and headaches.

These medicines include Slo-bid capsules and Uni-Dur and Uniphyl tablets.

The name of your medicine is: _______________.

Comment

- Convenient, since it can be given every 8 to 12 hours and is easy to take.
- Its major use is to boost the effect of daily preventer medicines (inhaled steroids, nedocromil or cromolyn).
- May cause gastric reflux.
- The usual dose may cause a toxic effect if you have a high fever, a virus infection or are taking certain medicines, including erythromycin.
- If you develop nausea, vomiting, a severe headache or become irritable, stop taking theophylline immediately. Then contact your doctor to discuss what changes should be made in your treatment plan.

Oral Steroids

Medicine type: Reliever

Decrease the inflammation of the lining of the windpipes.

Decrease the overreaction of the airways.

Decrease mucus production.

Improve the response of airways to adrenaline-like medicines.

Possible bad effects:

These are related to how much, how often, and how long the medicine is taken.

Steroids usually are taken for three to seven days, based on asthma signs or peak flow scores. After one day they may cause increased appetite, a feeling of well being, or problems sleeping. People who take oral steroids every day for more than two weeks may develop serious side effects.

You may be moody for a few days after you stop taking your steroid medicine.

These medicines include prednisone, prednisolone and methylprednisolone.

The name of your medicine is: _______________.

Comment

These steroids are *not* the muscle-building steroids that athletes use.

Name: Fred Mott

See back for instructions.

ASTHMA DIARY
PEAK FLOW

Please bring to each visit.

Triggers, Comments: First visit to specialist (8/25)

O - *Before bronchodilator*
X - *After bronchodilator*

Peak Flow Rate	Date	8/22	8/23	8/24	8/25	8/26	8/27	8/
100% 650								
Green Zone								
80% 520								
High Yellow Zone								
65% 420								
Low Yellow Zone								
50% 325								
Red Zone								

Medicines*	8/22	8/23	8/24	8/25	8/26	8/27	8/
Cromolyn or Nedocromil							
Aerobid 3 puffs 2x Inhaled steroid	✓✓	✓✓	✓✓	✓✓	✓✓	✓✓	✓✓
Proventil 2 puffs 2-4x Adrenaline-like medicine	✓✓✓	✓✓✓	✓✓✓✓	✓✓✓	✓✓✓	✓✓✓	✓✓✓
Prednisone 40mg 1x Oral steroid				✓	✓	✓	✓
Uniphyl 400mg 2x Theophylline	✓✓	✓✓	✓✓	✓✓	✓✓	✓✓	✓✓

Signs	8/22	8/23	8/24	8/25	8/26	8/27	8/
Wheeze	1	1	1	0	0	0	0
Cough	0	0	0	0	0	0	0
Activity	2	2	2	1	0	1	0
Sleep	2	2	2	0	0	0	0

* **Medicines:** • Cromolyn *(Intal)* • Nedocromil *(Tilade)* • Inhaled steroid *(Aerobid, Azmacort, Bec Pulmicort, Vanceril)* • Adrenaline-like medicine: albuterol *(Proventil, Ventolin)*, metaproterenol *(Maxair)*, terbutaline *(Brethaire or Bricanyl)* • Oral steroid *(prednisone, prednisolone, methylpredn (Slo-bid capsules, Uni-Dur and Uniphyl tablets).* Your doctor may prescribe others.

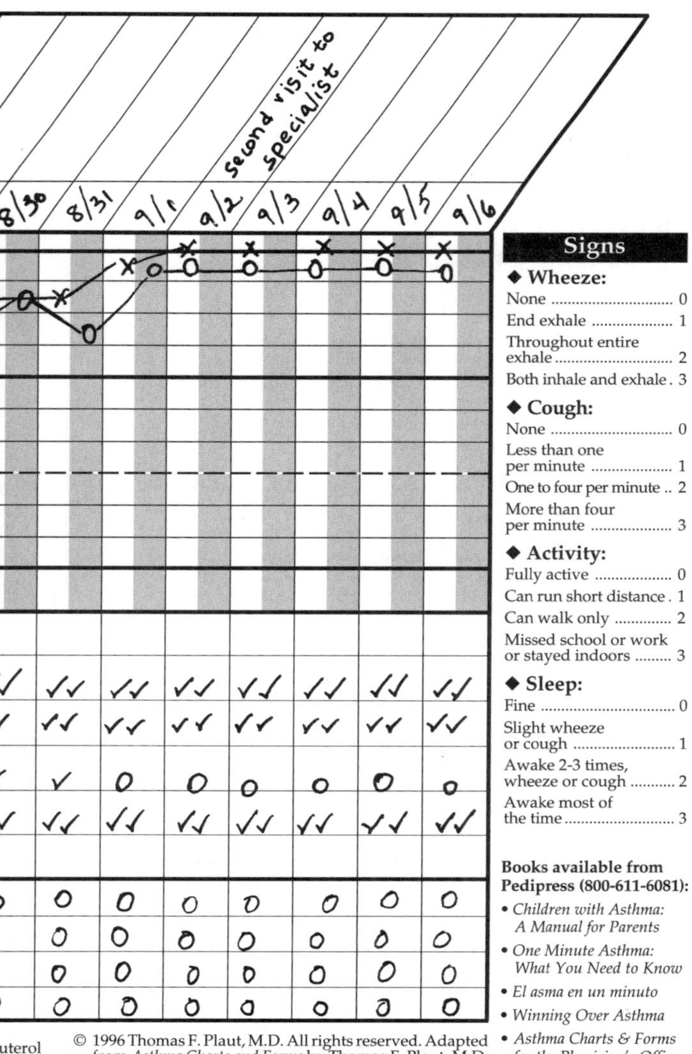

uterol
hylline

Signs

◆ Wheeze:
- None 0
- End exhale 1
- Throughout entire exhale 2
- Both inhale and exhale . 3

◆ Cough:
- None 0
- Less than one per minute 1
- One to four per minute .. 2
- More than four per minute 3

◆ Activity:
- Fully active 0
- Can run short distance . 1
- Can walk only 2
- Missed school or work or stayed indoors 3

◆ Sleep:
- Fine 0
- Slight wheeze or cough 1
- Awake 2-3 times, wheeze or cough 2
- Awake most of the time 3

Using the Asthma Diary

A well-designed asthma diary can help you learn how triggers and medicines affect your asthma. With this information, you and your doctor can work out a written plan that will help you care for your asthma at home.

Patients who use the asthma peak flow diary find it helps them to:

- Accurately recall events since the last visit.
- Learn when to start and reduce medicines.
- Communicate clearly and concisely on the telephone.
- Note the effects of changing a dosage or type of medicine.
- Determine the pattern of episodes caused by specific triggers.
- Identify triggers that provoke an episode.
- Remember to take or give medicines regularly.

Some children under the age of five can't blow peak flows reliably. They should use a diary that is based on the signs of asthma (see Asthma Signs Diary in the Resource Section).

Using the Home Treatment Plan

You need a written home treatment plan to remind you how to react to a drop in peak flow or the appearance of asthma signs and symptoms.

The easiest way to do this is to use a plan based on your peak flow zones. For each zone your doctor can write which medicine to take, how much and how often.

For children under five who don't blow peak flow well, base the home treatment plan on the Asthma Signs Diary (see Resource Section).

For Adults, Teens and Children Age 5 and Over
PEAK FLOW-BASED HOME TREATMENT PLAN

Name: Date: Best Peak Flow:

Green Zone

GREEN ZONE: Peak flow between ______ and ______.

- **Normal activity.**
  - ❑ Adrenaline-like medicine: albuterol *(Proventil, Ventolin)*, metaproterenol *(Alupent)*, pirbuterol *(Maxair)*, or terbutaline *(Brethaire or Bricanyl)*: 1 or 2 puffs 15 minutes before exercise.
  - ❑ Nedocromil *(Tilade)* or cromolyn *(Intal)*: 2 puffs before contact with cat or other allergen.
- **Medicine to be taken every day:**
  - ❑ Nedocromil *(Tilade)* or cromolyn *(Intal)*: ____ puffs____ times a day (a total of ____ puffs daily).
  - ❑ Inhaled steroid *(Aerobid, Azmacort, Beclovent, Flovent, Pulmicort, Vanceril)*: ____ puffs____ times a day (a total of ____ puffs daily).
  - ❑ Adrenaline-like medicine (see above): ____ puffs before each *nedocromil, cromolyn* or *inhaled steroid* dose for the first month.
  - ❑ Theophylline *(Slo-bid capsules, Uni-Dur and Uniphyl tablets)*: ____ mg ____ times a day.
  - ❑ Other:

High Yellow Zone

HIGH YELLOW ZONE: Peak flow between ______ and ______.

- **Eliminate triggers and add medicines. No strenuous exercise.**
- **Medicine to be taken:**
  - ❑ Adrenaline-like medicine (see above): ____ puffs by holding chamber. Take three to six times in 24 hours. Continue until peak flow is in the *Green Zone* for two days.
  - ❑ Double inhaled steroid (see above) to ____ puffs daily until peak flow is in the *Green Zone* for as long as it was in the *Yellow Zone*.

Low Yellow Zone

LOW YELLOW ZONE: Peak flow between ______ and ______.

Follow this plan if your peak flow does not reach the *High Yellow Zone* within 10 minutes after taking inhaled adrenaline-like medicine, or drops back into the *Low Yellow Zone* within four hours.

- ❑ Continue adrenaline-like medicine and yellow-zone medicines as above.
- ❑ Add oral steroid* _____ mg immediately. Continue each morning (8:00 A.M.) until peak flow is in the *Green Zone* for at least 24 hours.
- ❑ Please call the office before starting oral steroid.

* If your condition does not improve within two days after starting oral steroid, or if peak flow does not reach the *Green Zone* within seven days of treatment, see your doctor.

Red Zone

RED ZONE: Peak flow less than ______.

Follow this plan if peak flow does not reach *Low Yellow Zone* within 10 minutes after taking inhaled adrenaline-like medicine or drops back into *Red Zone* within four hours.

- ✓ Adrenaline-like medicine: ____ puffs by holding chamber.
- ✓ Give oral steroid ____ mg
- ✓ Visit your doctor or go to the Emergency Room.

 Pedipress, 125 Red Gate Lane, Amherst, MA 01002 publishes *Children with Asthma: A Manual for Parents, One Minute Asthma*, *El asma en un minuto*, *Winning Over Asthma* and *Asthma Charts & Forms for the Physician's Office*. (800) 611-6081.

Peak Flow Meter

The peak flow meter measures the fastest speed at which you can blow air out of your lungs.

During an asthma episode the windpipes begin to narrow slowly. This change can be measured with a peak flow meter.

The peak flow rate drops long before you or your doctor can hear any change with a stethoscope or see any sign of asthma.

If you learn to use a peak flow meter, you can start to treat your asthma very early at home. This will help you to avoid emergency care.

Almost all five-year-olds can learn to use a peak flow meter after they practice at home for a few weeks.

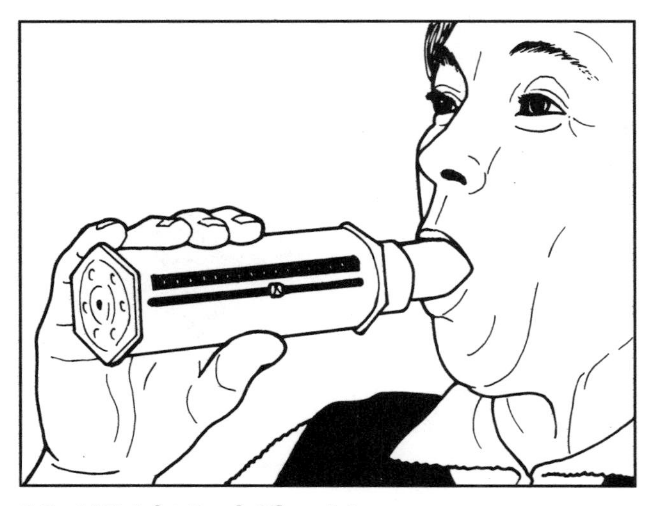

Mini-Wright Peak Flow Meter

Using a Peak Flow Meter

- Remove gum or food from your mouth, and move the pointer to zero.
- Stand up, and hold the meter horizontally with your fingers away from vent holes and the marker.
- Slowly breathe in as much air as you can with your mouth wide open.
- Put the mouthpiece on your tongue and close your lips snug around the mouthpiece.
- Blow out as fast as you can — a short sharp blast.
- Move the pointer to zero and wait at least ten seconds.
- Blow two more times.
- Mark your best score on your peak flow diary.

Note: If a peak flow attempt causes you to cough, this means your asthma is not adequately treated.

Peak Flow Zones

You and your doctor can create a plan to treat your asthma based on peak flow scores.

Your airways must be completely open with no swelling, no narrowing and no mucus, before you can determine your personal best peak flow.

Then, establish zones that match the colors of a traffic light.

Green-okay. Scores between 80 and 100 percent of your best score are in the green or okay zone. This means that air moves well through your windpipes.

Almost all patients will benefit from taking their preventer (anti-inflammatory) medicine every day, even when they are in the green zone and feeling fine. This treatment will greatly reduce the need for emergency care or hospitalization. It will prevent most signs, symptoms and episodes. The few problems that do occur will be much easier to treat.

Yellow-caution. Scores between 50 percent and 80 percent of your best score are in the yellow or caution zone.

Here you need to eliminate triggers and change your medicine routine according to your written plan.

Red-danger. If scores are less than 50 percent of your best peak flow, you need to see your doctor or go to the emergency room.

What is your best peak flow? ____________________

What is your green zone? ____________________

What is your yellow zone? ____________________

What is your red zone? ____________________

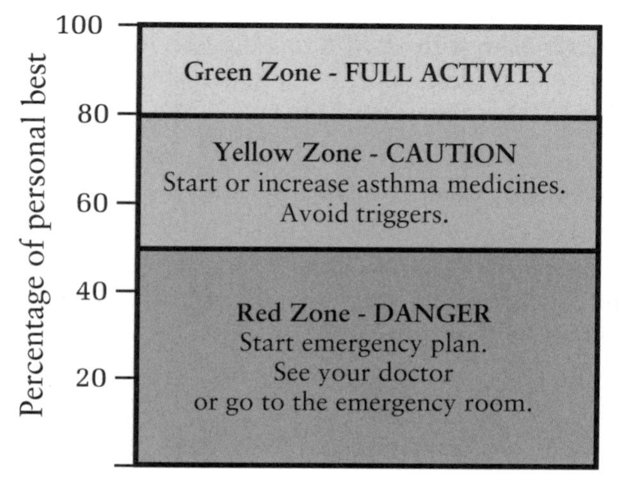

Peak Flow Zones

Getting Peak Flow Right

Blowing peak flow is like competing in the high jump. You count only the best of three tries. Do not average scores.

Your score may be falsely high if you:

- cough while blowing
- spit while blowing. This problem is seen when using a small mouthpiece.

Your score may be falsely low if:

- you blow too slow
- you don't hold your lips snug around the mouthpiece
- your fingers block a vent or they block the marker.

Never blame a low peak flow score on poor technique or poor effort. If your technique is poor on one blow you should be able to correct it on the next. If your effort is poor you should be able to increase your score at the next blow.

If you are tired and can only blow a peak flow in the red zone you probably have a serious problem and should see a doctor right away.

If you are unable to move the marker or it hardly moves call 911 immediately and go to the emergency room.

How to Use an Inhaler (MDI)

Effective use of the metered-dose inhaler (MDI) depends on proper position and timing.

- Hold the mouthpiece one or two inches from your lips and open your mouth wide.
- Start to breathe in and then squeeze the little medicine can down.
- Breathe in slowly for three to five seconds.
- Hold your breath as long as possible up to 10 seconds.
- Wait 30 seconds before taking another puff.
- To increase effect during an episode, wait one to three minutes between puffs of adrenaline-like medicine.

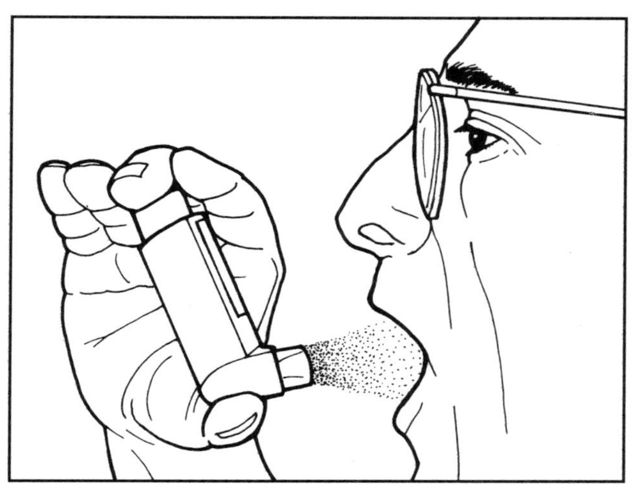

Proper Inhaler Position

Holding Chamber

A holding chamber helps you use an inhaler effectively because it:

- Is easy to hold in the right position.
- Holds the puff of medicine so you can inhale it slowly.
- Helps more medicine get to the windpipes where it works.
- Lessens the bad taste of the medicine.
- Reduces possible bad effects of medicine.

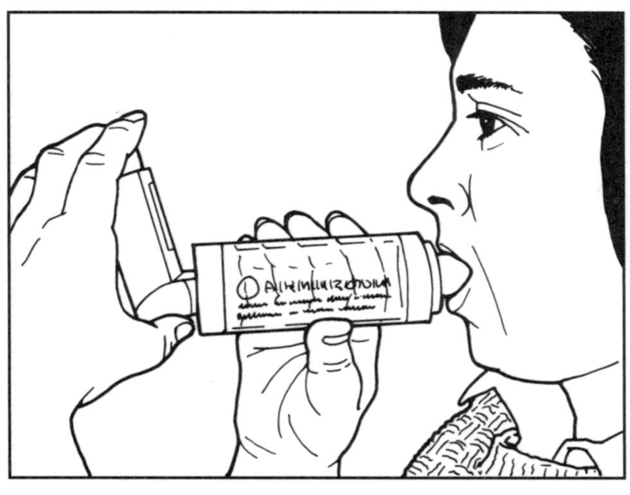

Aerochamber Holding Chamber

Using a Holding Chamber

- Remove the cap from your inhaler.
- Place the mouthpiece on your tongue.
- Close your lips snugly around the mouthpiece.
- Spray one puff of medicine into the chamber.
- Breathe in slowly taking three to five seconds.
- Hold your breath for 10 seconds.
- Remove the chamber from your mouth and breathe out.

If you cannot hold your breath for 10 seconds, hold it for five seconds. Then breathe out, keeping your lips snug around the mouthpiece. Breathe in slowly and hold your breath again for five seconds.

Wait at least 30 seconds between each new puff of medicine. Your doctor will tell you how many puffs of medicine to take and which medicine to take first.

Never put two puffs in the chamber at the same time since this *reduces* the actual amount delivered.

To increase effect during an episode, wait one to three minutes between puffs of adrenaline-like medicine.

Compressor-Driven Nebulizer (Mist Machine)

Use a nebulizer if you are too sick to use a holding chamber.

Treatment should be given every _____ hours. Treatment should take 4 to 12 minutes, depending on the efficiency of your nebulizer cup. If you do not get much better in 12 minutes or if symptoms come back in less than four hours, your treatment plan is not satisfactory and needs to be changed.

To Set-Up:

- Measure ______ cc of normal saline or cromolyn and put it into the plastic cup.
- Measure ______ cc of ______________ and put it into the plastic cup with the saline or cromolyn. Once you know the number of drops, you can count them as a check.
- If you use a single unit dose, just put it in the plastic cup.
- For best effect use a mouthpiece. A mask may be useful for some very young patients. Pointing the mouthpiece at the patient, the "blow by" technique, delivers much less medicine to the lungs.

The medicine mist must settle in your windpipes in order to work. To aid this process:

- Breathe slowly, 10 to 20 times a minute, if possible.
- Take longer to breathe in than to breathe out, if possible.

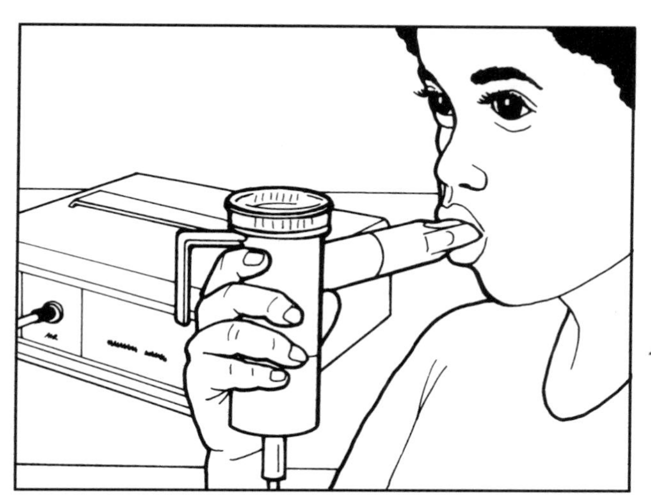

ProNeb Compressor-Driven Nebulizer

Antihistamines

Postnasal drip can trigger a cough.

This cough may lead to asthma symptoms.

Antihistamines may dry the nasal passages and reduce swelling and postnasal drip. When the drip stops, asthma symptoms often improve.

Why does the antihistamine package warn people with asthma not to use this medicine?

Doctors used to think that antihistamines would dry the mucus in the windpipes and make it harder to cough up, but this has not been proven.

It is safe for people with asthma to take antihistamines.

Cough Medicines

Should a patient with asthma take cough medicine?

Coughing with exercise or at night is a sign of poor asthma control.

Report this coughing to your doctor so that you can adjust your asthma treatment plan.

If the cough continues *after* your asthma is fully treated, a cough medicine may be helpful.

Which Inhaler Should You Use First?

If you take more than one medicine by inhaler, be sure to use the reliever medicine (that dilates the windpipes) first.

Reliever medicines go by the generic names of albuterol (Proventil and Ventolin), metaproterenol (Alupent), pirbuterol (Maxair) and terbutaline (Brethaire and Bricanyl).

The reliever medicine will open the windpipes so that cromolyn, nedocromil or inhaled steroids can get deep into the windpipes where they work.

Is Your Inhaler Empty?

Metered-Dose Inhaler (MDI). You can figure out how many days a full MDI will last. To do this, divide the number of puffs you take each day into the total number of puffs in the canister. (It is written on the label.) For example, if you take eight puffs each day from a 200-puff canister, it will last 25 days. Write this "discard date" on the canister.

We no longer recommend other ways of checking an MDI (the puff test, the shake test and the float test) because they are less accurate and may waste medicine. Floating cromolyn or nedocromil inhalers will cause their valves to plug.

Asthma Stories

The Light Bulb

Do you call an electrician when a light bulb burns out?

You can change the bulb yourself.

Do you call a doctor when you have an asthma episode?

- If you have worked out a written plan with your doctor, you can take care of most asthma problems at home.

The Runner

One of my twelve-year-old patients runs the half mile. Her coach thought she was very good.

After she started to use her albuterol inhaler before running, he realized she was excellent.

- Pretreatment may allow you to compete at a higher level.

Fighting Asthma

Suppose your house is on fire.

Do you want the firefighters to squirt a little water on it and then wait to see if the fire goes out?

Suppose you have an asthma attack.

Do you want to use a little medicine and wait to see if the attack stops?

- Intensive treatment will control an attack faster.

The Umbrella

When it rains, an umbrella can keep you dry. If you close it while it is still raining, you will get wet.

Asthma "preventer" medicines work like an umbrella. They protect you from symptoms and episodes.

- Problems often return if you stop the preventer medicine.

Resource Section

Pedipress Books

Pedipress, Inc.
125 Red Gate Lane
Amherst, MA 01002
Toll free: (800) 611-6081
Fax: (800) 499-6464
Call for quantity discount.

Children with Asthma: A Manual for Parents
Thomas F. Plaut, M.D.

Pocket-size, 304 pages, 1995; $10.00. Full-size, 296 pages plus 1995 supplement, $14.95.

Known as "the asthma bible," *Children with Asthma* emphasizes the importance of the parent's role in asthma management. It teaches the basics of asthma, how medicines work, and when to call for help. Has sections on infants, children and teenagers. Applies to adults as well. Contains stories by parents as well as illustrations, tables and instructions. The 1995 supplement outlines the major changes in asthma care since 1988, including new techniques for treatment, new devices, new diaries, and new home treatment plans.

One Minute Asthma
Thomas F. Plaut, M.D.
48 pages, 1996, $5.00

Accurate, clear and easy to read. Covers the basics of asthma and the medicines used to treat it. An ideal book for people starting to learn about asthma: patients, parents, teachers, coaches, friends, relatives, and baby-sitters. Illustrated.

El asma en un minuto
Thomas F. Plaut, M.D.
40 pages, 1995, $4.95

Spanish edition of *One Minute Asthma*. Similar contents.

Winning Over Asthma
Eileen Dolan Silk
40 pages, 2nd Edition, 1996, $7.00

This picture book presents asthma facts while telling the story of five-year-old Graham. It describes the asthma reaction, mentions several triggers and medicines, and emphasizes team work between parents and physician. Illustrates that childhood asthma can be controlled.

Asthma Peak Flow Diary
Thomas F. Plaut, M.D.
Three colors, pad of 100 sheets, $10.00

An ideal learning and monitoring tool for patients and parents who want to understand and control asthma.

Asthma Signs Diary
Thomas F. Plaut, M.D.
Three colors, pad of 50 sheets, $7.50

Helps parents learn about and control asthma in children under five years of age.

Asthma Charts & Forms for the Physician's Office
Thomas F. Plaut, M.D. and Carla Brennan.
64 pages with IBM/PC or Macintosh disk, $75.00

Revised 1995. Charts, diaries, questionnaires and letters that increase efficiency, save time and improve patient compliance.

Organizations

National Asthma Education and Prevention Program
4733 Bethesda Avenue, Suite 530
Bethesda, MD 20814-4820

(301) 251-1222

Distributes the Executive Summary of the NHLBI *Guidelines for the Diagnosis and Management of Asthma* free to the public. This 40-page book is the most up-to-date reference on current asthma treatment. The NAEPP provides information for patients, health professionals, schools and the public.

Asthma and Allergy Foundation of America
1125 15th Street., N.W., Suite 502
Washington, DC 20005

(202) 466-7643
(800) 7-ASTHMA

A number of chapters throughout the country offer support groups, school programs, community workshops, conferences, and the Asthma Care Training program.

National Allergy and Asthma Network/Mothers of Asthmatics
3554 Chain Bridge Road, Suite 200
Fairfax, VA 22030-2709

(703) 385-4403
(800) 878-4403

Provides information for the parents of children with asthma through *MA Report* (a newsletter), booklets and videos.

American Association for Respiratory Care
11030 Ables Lane
Dallas, TX 75229

(214) 243-2272

National organization of respiratory therapists. Offers a free, peak flow-based program for schools, *Peak Performance, USA*.

American Lung Association
1740 Broadway
New York, NY 10019

(800) LUNG-USA

More than 300 local and state lung associations provide many asthma education services. Some chapters sponsor support groups, newsletters and asthma camps.

American College of Allergy and Immunology
85 West Algonquin Road, Suite 550
Arlington Heights, IL 60005

(708) 427-1200
(800) 842-7777

Provides educational materials and forms for use in schools. Sponsors regional asthma education conferences for the public.

National Jewish Center for Immunology and Respiratory Disease
1400 Jackson Street
Denver, CO 80206

(800) 222-LUNG

Provides information on asthma and lung disease via the toll-free LUNG LINE, (800) 222-LUNG. Engaged in treatment, research and education in chronic respiratory diseases. Accepts patients by physician and self-referral.

Food Allergy Network
10400 Eaton Place, Ste 107
Fairfax, VA 22030-5674

(703) 691-3179
(800) 929-4040

Provides information on food allergy to patients, health professionals and the public through a newsletter, videos and cookbooks.

American Academy of Allergy and Immunology
611 East Wells Street
Milwaukee, WI 53202

(414) 272-6071
(800) 822-2762

Pamphlets on asthma, allergies, mold and pollen.

Newsletter

Asthma Update
David Jamison, Editor
123 Monticello Avenue, Suite B
Annapolis, MD 21401

(410) 267-8329

Quarterly newsletter for parents and adult patients. Includes annotated abstracts from current medical journals. Four pages per issue. $12.00 per year.

About the Author

Thomas F. Plaut, M.D., has cared for thousands of children with asthma. He is a nationally known asthma specialist and the author of *Children with Asthma: A Manual for Parents*, *One Minute Asthma: What You Need to Know*, and *Asthma Charts & Forms for the Physician's Office.* He serves as an asthma consultant to HMOs, physicians and health organizations.

He is on the editorial board of *Advance for Managers of Respiratory Care* and is the medical consultant to *Asthma Update*, a newsletter for patients and professionals. His office is in Amherst, Massachusetts.

Acknowledgments

Sincere thanks to the following for their useful comments: Arthur Bergner, M.D., Gary Brecher, M.D., Ellie Goldberg, M.Ed., Jean Hanson, R.N., M.N., Andrew Larkin, M.D., Guillermo Mendoza, M.D., Shirley Murphy, M.D., Michael T. Newhouse, M.D., Jane Purser, M.D., Jackie Trovato, Jeffrey Wald, M.D., Paul Walker, M.D. and Michael Welch, M.D.

Order Form

_______ ***Children with Asthma: A Manual for Parents***
1995. 304 pages, pocket-size. Single copy $10.00 or ten copies $80.00.

_______ ***Children with Asthma: A Manual for Parents***
296 pages, full-size with 1995 supplement. Single copy $14.95 or 10 copies $120.00.

_______ ***One Minute Asthma: What You Need to Know***
48 pages. Single copy $5.00 or ten copies $20.00.

_______ ***El asma en un minuto***
Spanish-language version of *One Minute Asthma*, 40 pages. Single copy $4.95 or ten copies $20.00.

_______ ***Winning Over Asthma***
40 pages. Single copy $7.00 or ten copies $55.00.

_______ ***Asthma Peak Flow Diary***
3 colors, pad of 100 sheets $10.00 or ten pads $90.00.

_______ ***Asthma Signs Diary***
3 colors, pad of 50 sheets $7.50 or ten pads $60.00.

Minimum order $20.00. Add $5.00 for shipping within the 48 contiguous states. For orders over $150.00, add 5% of the total order. Please call for shipping costs to other locations.

Name _______________________________

Street _______________________________

City ____________________ State _____ Zip ________

❑ Mastercard ❑ Visa # ______________________

Exp. Date __________ Signature ______________________

Send check or money order to:

Pedipress Fulfillment Center
200 State Road
So. Deerfield, MA 01373

Phone: 800-611-6081; Fax: 800-499-6464